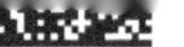

21 No-Cook Dinner Recipes to Help Reduce Inflammation

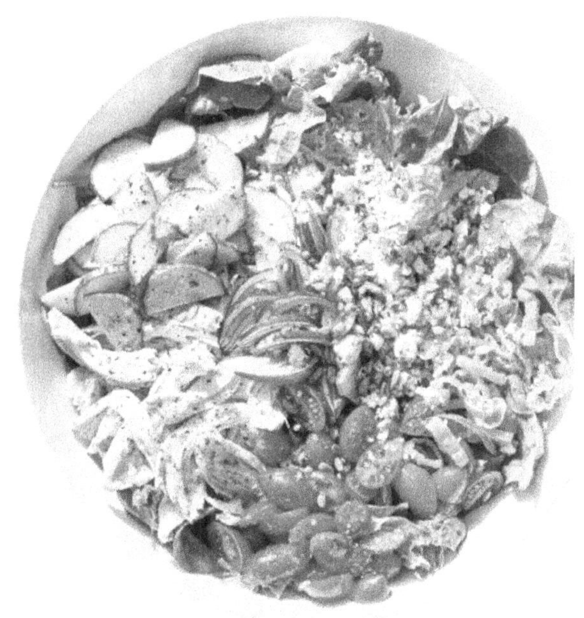

Dr. Malvin Harison

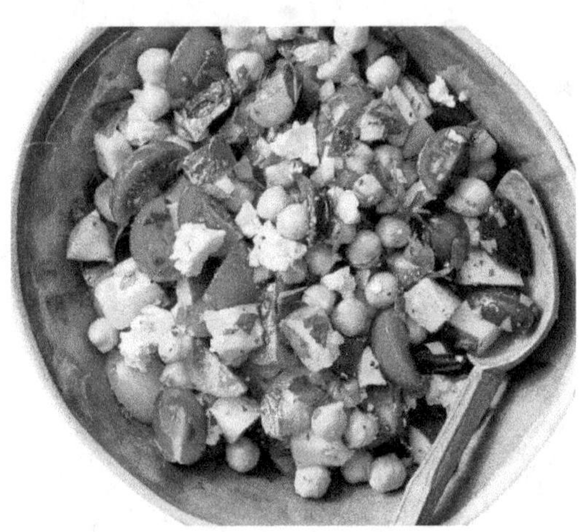

TABLE OF CONTENT

Keep the oven or broiler perfect and cool with these delectable and sound no-cook supper recipes. To make one of these invigorating dishes, you just have to utilize pre-cooked, canned, or new fixings. In addition, they're loaded with mitigating food varieties like avocados, chickpeas, and salmon to assist you with battling annoying side effects of aggravation like weakness, trouble resting, and stomach-related issues. Recipes like our Salmon and Avocado Jab Bowl and Hacked Salad with Chickpeas, Olives, and Feta are supporting dinners that will help you and your kitchen cool down and remain feeling your best this mid-year.

21 No-Cook Dinner Recipes to Help Reduce Inflammation

1. Chopped Power Salad with Chicken

Partake in this filling and vivid plate of mixed greens for lunch or supper. The dressing gets made in the very bowl that the serving of mixed greens is thrown in, so the greens retain all of the flavor.

What Supplements Does This Recipe Give?
This recipe has some great nourishment details. One serving of this power salad will give you around 14% of your everyday fiber, 23% of your potassium for the afternoon, very nearly a day of protein, and an excess of vitamin A.

Is This Recipe Without Gluten?
Yes. Since this recipe utilizes no fixings containing gluten, it is without gluten.

Is This a Low-Carb Recipe?
Indeed, this is a low-carb, high-protein recipe.

Is Green-Leaf Lettuce Sound?
Contrasted with its dim green partners (hi, spinach and kale!) green-leaf lettuce doesn't have as much nourishment, however, it adds a L-ascorbic acid to your plate.

Tips from the Test Kitchen

I Don't Have Green-Leaf Lettuce, Could I at any point Utilize Another Sort?

Absolutely! Green-leaf lettuce is a sort of free-leaf lettuce, which has inexactly clustered leaves rather than tight heads. It has a gentle, sweet flavor with a marginally fresh and delicate surface. On the off chance that you can't find green-leaf lettuce, you can utilize red-leaf, butterhead, Little Diamond, or romaine.

Can I at any point Utilize Rotisserie Chicken?

Indeed, you can. If you're restricting your sodium or immersed fat admission, you might need to leave out the skin while destroying the rotisserie chicken. You can likewise prepare or bubble chicken bosoms and shred them, or utilize extra meal chicken from a past recipe.

Is There a Substitute for Pepperoncini?

Pepperoncini peppers are commonly salted and are gentle and tart in flavor. You can substitute them with cut-cured banana peppers, which have a comparatively fiery flavor and fresh surface.

What Is a Slashed Serving of Mixed Greens?

In a hacked salad, the fixings are all cleaved into more modest scaled-down pieces. The fixings can either be formed, have significance, they're organized on a platter, or thrown along with the dressing. Hacked plates of mixed greens have a more reliable surface and the fixings are very much conveyed for each chomp.

Fixings

¼ cup extra-virgin olive oil

3 tablespoons lemon juice

1 clove garlic, ground

½ teaspoon dried oregano

½ teaspoon sugar

¼ teaspoon salt

¼ teaspoon ground pepper

4 cups torn green-leaf lettuce

4 cups child spinach

2 cups destroyed cooked chicken

1 cup divided grape tomatoes

1 cup divided and cut cucumber

½ cup fragmented red onion

⅓ cup cut pepperoncini

⅓ cup disintegrated feta cheddar

2 tablespoons toasted unsalted sunflower seeds

Headings

Whisk oil, lemon juice, garlic, oregano, sugar, salt, and pepper together in an enormous bowl. Put lettuce, spinach, chicken, tomatoes, cucumber, onion, and pepperoncini; throw to cover. Sprinkled with feta, sunflower seeds and served.

2. Salmon and Avocado Jab Bowl

Poke (articulated poh-kay), the scaled-down marinated fish salad well known in Hawaii, is famous to such an extent that it's sold by the pound in grocery stores. Presently it has crossed the Pacific to turn into the dinner in a bowl of the day, served in restaurants from Los Angeles to New York. Be that as it may, it's not difficult to make at home with this speedy recipe. Sriracha and Chinese-style mustard add a hint of intensity to the exemplary jab preparation of soy sauce and sesame oil. Serving it over an earthy-colored rice salad makes it a dinner.

Fixings

Poke

1 pound of recently frozen wild salmon, cleaned and cut into 3/4-inch solid shapes

1 medium ready avocado, diced

½ cup daintily cut yellow onion

½ cup meagerly cut scallion greens

½ cup cleaved new cilantro

¼ cup of tobiko (flying fish roe) or other caviar

3 tablespoons decreased sodium tamari

2 teaspoons toasted (dull) sesame oil

½ teaspoon Sriracha

Colored Rice Salad

2 cups cooked short-grain earthy colored rice, warmed

2 cups stuffed hot greens, like arugula, watercress or mizuna

2 tablespoons rice vinegar

2 tablespoons extra-virgin olive oil

1 tablespoon Chinese-style or Dijon mustard

Bearings

Tenderly consolidate salmon, avocado, onion, scallion greens, cilantro, tobiko (or caviar), tamari, sesame oil, and Sriracha in a medium bowl.

Join rice and greens in an enormous bowl. Whisk vinegar, oil, and mustard in a little bowl. Add to the rice salad and blend well. Serve the jab on the rice salad.

3. Caprese Sandwich

This caprese sandwich is straight from the basil and good from thick, dried-up crusty bread. The sun-dried tomatoes develop the flavor. Finishing off the bread with a layer of basil leaves and utilizing toasted bread assists with holding the sandwich back from getting soaked on the off chance that you want to make it a couple of hours to come.

Fixings

2 cups crusty bread, toasted

¼ cup delicately pressed new basil leaves

2 ounces mozzarella cheddar, cut

2 cuts tomato

1 tablespoon hacked sun-dried tomatoes in oil

1 teaspoon balsamic coating

Headings

Top 1 crusty bread cut with half of the basil leaves; top with mozzarella, tomato, and sun-dried tomatoes. Sprinkle with balsamic coating and top with the leftover basil leaves and crusty bread cut. Slice down the middle slantingly and serve.

4. Chopped Salad with Chickpeas, Olives and Feta

This fast and simple hacked salad is roused by the kinds of the Mediterranean, including chickpeas, cucumber, and feta. A garlicky oil and vinegar dressing unites everything.

Fixings

2 tablespoons extra-virgin olive oil

2 tablespoons red wine vinegar

¼ teaspoon garlic powder

¼ teaspoon salt

¼ teaspoon ground pepper

1 (15 ounces) can no-salt-added chickpeas, washed

1 cup diced cucumber

1 cup quartered cherry tomatoes

⅓ cup hacked parsley

¼ cup finely hacked red onion

¼ cup split Kalamata olives

¼ cup disintegrated feta

Bearings

Whisk oil, vinegar, garlic powder, salt, and pepper in a huge bowl. Add chickpeas, cucumber, tomatoes, parsley, onion, olives, and feta; throw to cover.

5. Tuna poke

Jab (articulated jab ay), a Hawaiian word signifying "to cleave" or "to cut," alludes to a customary Hawaiian serving of mixed greens of diced crude fish in a straightforward, soy-based sauce with punchy flavors like toasted sesame and hacked scallion greens. These fish jab bowls highlight prepared earthy-colored rice and new veggies for a sound, fulfilling dinner loaded with protein and fiber.

Fixings

¾ cup meagerly cut scallion greens

¼ cup diminished sodium tamari

1 ½ tablespoons mirin

1 ½ tablespoons toasted (dim) sesame oil

1 tablespoon toasted sesame seeds

2 teaspoons ground new ginger

½ teaspoon squashed red pepper (Discretionary)

12 ounces sushi-grade fish, cleaned and cut into 1/2-inch blocks

2 cups cooked earthy colored rice

2 tablespoons rice vinegar

2 cups cut snow peas

2 cups cut cucumber

¼ cup hacked chives

1/4 cup furikake preparing

Bearings

Whisk scallion greens, tamari, mirin, oil, sesame seeds, ginger, and squashed red pepper, if utilized, in a medium bowl. Put away 2 tablespoons of the sauce in a little bowl. Add fish to the sauce in the medium bowl and tenderly throw to cover.

6. Salmon-Stuffed Avocados

Canned salmon is an important storeroom staple and a functional method for including heart-solid, omega-3-rich fish in your eating regimen. Here, we consolidate it with avocados in a simple no-cook dinner.

Fixings

½ cup nonfat plain Greek yogurt

½ cup diced celery

2 tablespoons hacked new parsley

1 tablespoon lime juice

2 teaspoons mayonnaise

1 teaspoon Dijon mustard

⅛ teaspoon salt

⅛ teaspoon ground pepper

2 (5 ounces) jars of salmon, depleted, chipped, skin and bones eliminated
2 avocados
Cleaved chives for embellish
Bearings
Consolidate yogurt, celery, parsley, lime juice, mayonnaise, mustard, salt, and pepper in a medium bowl; blend well. Add salmon and blend well.

Divide avocados longwise and eliminate pits. Scoop around 1 tablespoon of tissue from every avocado half into a little bowl. Pound the scooped-out avocado tissue with a fork and mix it into the salmon combination.

Fill every avocado half with around 1/4 cup of the salmon blend, mounding it on top of the avocado parts. Decorate with chives, whenever you want.

7. Avocado Fish Salad

Spice up a jar of fish with this simple avocado fish salad recipe. Luxurious avocado adds a smoothness that is cut with a hit of corrosiveness from lemon and a briny punch from feta cheddar. Romaine hearts and cucumber offer a reviving crunch.

Fixings

3 tablespoons extra-virgin olive oil

2 tablespoons lemon juice

¼ teaspoon salt

2 medium avocados, cleaved (around 2 1/2 cups)

2 (5-ounce) jars of strong white fish in oil, depleted and chipped

4 cups romaine hearts

1 cup cleaved English cucumber

⅓ cup disintegrated feta cheddar

¼ cup toasted cut almonds

¼ cup cleaved pitted Kalamata olives

3 tablespoons slashed new-level leaf parsley

Headings

Whisk oil, lemon squeeze, and salt together in an enormous bowl; add avocados and throw delicately to completely cover. Add fish, romaine, cucumber, feta, almonds, olives, and parsley to the avocado combination; throw delicately to consolidate. Serve right away or refrigerate for as long as 60 minutes.

8. Tofu poke

This quick vegetarian rendition of jab (the conventional Hawaiian serving of mixed greens of diced crude fish thrown in a soy-sesame sauce) trades in extra-firm tofu for fish while stacking your bowl with vegetables and crunchy clinchers like pea shoots and peanuts. Serve over earthy-colored rice rather than the zucchini noodles to add a generous increase in fiber.

Fixings

¾ cup meagerly cut scallion greens

¼ cup diminished sodium tamari

1 ½ tablespoons mirin

1 ½ tablespoons toasted (dim) sesame oil

1 tablespoon toasted sesame seeds

2 teaspoons ground new ginger

½ teaspoon squashed red pepper (Discretionary)

1 (12 ounces) bundle of extra-firm tofu, depleted and cut into 1/2-inch pieces

4 cups zucchini noodles

2 tablespoons rice vinegar

2 cups destroyed carrots

2 cups pea shoots

¼ cup toasted slashed peanuts

¼ cup slashed new basil

Headings

Whisk scallion greens, tamari, mirin, oil, sesame seeds, ginger, and squashed red pepper, if utilized, in a medium bowl. Put away 2 tablespoons of the sauce in a little bowl. Add tofu to the sauce in the medium bowl and tenderly throw to cover.

Join zucchini noodles and vinegar in an enormous bowl. Split between 4 dishes and top each with 3/4 cup tofu, 1/2 cup carrots, and pea shoots, and 1 tablespoon every peanuts and basil. Sprinkle with the held sauce and serve.

9. Green Goddess Sandwich

This green goddess sandwich is a new and fulfilling sandwich. The dressing sneaks up all of a sudden with tricks and lemon juice. The cucumber and fledglings add a pleasant crunch, and the carefully prepared avocado gets the richness.

Fixings

½ cup plain entire milk stressed yogurt, like Greek-style

½ cup hacked new parsley leaves

2 tablespoons hacked new tarragon leaves

2 tablespoons hacked new chives

1 tablespoon tricks, washed and slashed

1 clove garlic, ground

1 ½ teaspoons ground lemon zing

¼ cup lemon juice

1 medium avocado, cut into 8 cuts

¼ teaspoon salt

4 cuts generous entire wheat bread (1/2-inch)

1 cup watercress or spinach, isolated

1 cup meagerly cut cucumber, partitioned

½ cup horse feed sprouts, partitioned

Headings

Join yogurt, parsley, tarragon, chives, escapades, garlic, lemon zing, and 2 tablespoons of lemon juice in a medium bowl; race until very much blended.

Sprinkle avocado uniformly with salt and the excess 2 tablespoons lemon juice.

Spread 2 piling tablespoons of the yogurt blend on each bread cut. Top every one of 2 bread cuts with 1/2 cup watercress and cucumber,

4 cuts of avocado, and 1/4 cup hay sprouts. Top with the leftover 2 bread cuts, spread-side down. Slice down the middle and serve right away.

10. Avocado Fish Spinach Salad

Avocado adds smoothness while sunflower seeds give surface and smash in this simple fish spinach salad.

Fixings

½ (5 ounce) can water-pressed fish

¼ cup diced avocado

¼ cup divided cherry tomatoes

1 ½ tablespoons poppy seed dressing

1 tablespoon diced red onion

1 tablespoon extra-virgin olive oil

2 cups child spinach

1 tablespoon sunflower seeds

Headings

Join fish, avocado, tomatoes, dressing, onion, and oil in a medium bowl. Serve over spinach and sprinkle with sunflower seeds.

11. Cucumber Chickpea Salad with Feta and Lemon

This recipe is tart and invigorating. You can enjoy it all alone or add some greens for a simple lunch or supper. We love the green kind of dill, however, another new spice like oregano, parsley, or chives will function admirably in its place.

Fixings

2 tablespoons extra-virgin olive oil

2 tablespoons lemon juice

¼ teaspoon salt

¼ teaspoon ground pepper

1 15-ounce can of chickpeas, washed

2 cups diced cucumber

⅓ cup disintegrated feta cheddar

¼ cup finely hacked red onion

¼ cup diced red chime pepper

2 tablespoons hacked new dill

Bearings

Mix oil, lemon squeeze, salt, and pepper together in a huge bowl. Add chickpeas, cucumber, feta, red onion, ringer pepper, and dill; throw to cover.

12. Brown Rice Shrimp Bowl, Tomatoes & Avocado

This speedy and simple bowl matches earthy-colored rice with cooked shrimp, thrown in a ginger-soy-sesame sauce, to make a tasty dish in a matter of moments. Finishing off with tomatoes and avocado adds tone and supplements. Go through extra earthy-colored rice or pick a bundle of pre-cooked earthy-colored rice from the supermarket to keep this dinner no-cook.

Fixings

¾ cup daintily cut scallion greens

¼ cup decreased sodium tamari

1 ½ tablespoons mirin

1 ½ tablespoons toasted (dull) sesame oil

1 tablespoon white sesame seeds

2 teaspoons ground new ginger

½ teaspoon squashed red pepper (Discretionary)

12 ounces of cooked shrimp, slice into 1/2-inch pieces

2 cups cooked earthy colored rice

2 tablespoons rice vinegar

2 cups cut cherry tomatoes

2 cups diced avocado

¼ cup cleaved cilantro

¼ cup toasted dark sesame seeds
Bearings
Whisk scallion greens, tamari, mirin, oil, white sesame seeds, ginger, and squashed red pepper, if utilized, in a medium bowl. Put away 2 tablespoons of the sauce in a little bowl. Add shrimp to the sauce in the medium bowl and delicately throw to cover.

Join rice and vinegar in an enormous bowl. Split between 4 dishes and top each with 3/4 cup shrimp, 1/2 cup every tomato and avocado, and 1 tablespoon every cilantro and dark sesame seeds. Sprinkle with the held sauce and serve.

13. Chicken Caesar Salad Wraps

These chicken Caesar salad wraps make for a fast, simple lunch or supper. We like a blend of romaine and kale for surface and variety, yet you can utilize either in the event that you like. Romaine won't hold well once dressed, so we prescribe making this envelope as long as 1 day in advance or the leaves will get spongy. Parmesan crisps go about as another bread garnish-like component — utilize locally acquired crisps or make your own with our Parmesan Crisps recipe.

Fixings

5 cups cleaved romaine lettuce hearts and additional lacinato kale

2 cups cleaved cooked chicken bosom

½ cup packaged yogurt-based Caesar dressing

2 tablespoons ground Parmesan cheddar

½ cup garlic-and-cheddar prepared bread garnishes, coarsely squashed

¼ cup Parmesan crisps coarsely squashed

4 (10-inch) entire wheat tortillas

Headings

Join romaine (or potentially kale), chicken, dressing, and ground Parmesan in an enormous bowl; throw to cover. In the case of utilizing kale, rub the dressing into the leaves to soften. Overlay bread garnishes and Parmesan crisps into the serving of mixed greens blend.

Lay 1 tortilla on a cutting board. Spoon 1 1/2 cups of salad blend into the focal point of the tortilla; roll up like a burrito. Slice down the middle, whenever you want. Rehash with the leftover tortillas and salad combination.

Tip

Find yogurt-based Caesar dressing, for example, Bolthouse Ranches, in the produce part of the supermarket.

14. Nut Zoodles with Edamame

A bundle of new zucchini noodles gets thrown with shelled edamame and locally acquired nut sauce in these 5-minute, no-cook vegetable noodle bowls. Since arranged sauces and dressings are usually high in sodium, filter the mark and settle on those that contain 150 mg sodium or less per tablespoon.

Fixings

1 (12-ounce) bundle of new zucchini noodles

1 cup frozen shelled edamame, defrosted

⅓ cup Thai-style nut sauce or dressing

Headings

Join zucchini noodles and edamame in a huge bowl.

Top with nut sauce (or dressing) and throw delicately until very much covered; split between 2 dishes.

To make ahead
Refrigerate for as long as 1 day.

15. 3-Fixing Green Goddess White Bean Salad

Stowed salad and slaw mixes are incredible alternate route elements for changing it up without expecting to wash and cleave heaps of various vegetables. Prepare a kale-and-broccoli slaw blend in with canned white beans and yogurt-based green goddess dressing for a crunchy primary dish salad in minutes.

Fixings

1 (10-ounce) sack kale-and-broccoli slaw blend

1 (15 ounces) can no-salt-added cannellini beans, washed

¼ cup green goddess yogurt dressing

Bearings

Throw slaw blend in with beans.

Add dressing and throw to cover.

To make ahead
Refrigerate salad (Stage 1) for as long as 1 day.
Throw with dressing not long prior to eating.

16. Mediterranean Chickpea Salad

Fixings:

2 cups canned chickpeas, depleted and washed

1 cup cherry tomatoes, split

1 cucumber, diced

1/2 red onion, finely hacked

1/4 cup Kalamata olives, hollowed and cut

1/4 cup feta cheddar, disintegrated (discretionary)

2 tablespoons extra-virgin olive oil

2 tablespoons new lemon juice

1 teaspoon dried oregano

Salt and pepper to taste

New parsley for decorating

Guidelines:

In an enormous bowl, join chickpeas, cherry tomatoes, cucumber, red onion, and olives.

In a little bowl, whisk together olive oil, lemon juice, dried oregano, salt, and pepper.

Pour the dressing over the plate of mixed greens and throw to join.

Whenever wanted, sprinkle with feta cheddar and trim with new parsley.

Serve chilled.

17. Avocado and Salmon Wraps

Fixings:

2 huge entire grain tortillas

1 ready avocado, daintily cut

4 oz smoked salmon

1/4 cup Greek yogurt

1 tablespoon new dill, hacked

1 tablespoon tricks

Juice of 1/2 lemon

Salt and pepper to taste

Child spinach leaves

Directions:

Spread out the tortillas and layer with avocado cuts and smoked salmon.

In a little bowl, blend Greek yogurt, dill, tricks, lemon squeeze, salt, and pepper to make the sauce.

Spread the sauce over the salmon.

Add a small bunch of child spinach leaves on top.

Roll up the tortillas firmly and cut down the middle askew.

Serve right away.

18. Quinoa and Dark Bean Salad

Fixings:

1 cup cooked quinoa, cooled

1 cup canned dark beans, depleted and washed

1 cup corn pieces (new or frozen, defrosted)

1 red chime pepper, diced

1/2 cup new cilantro, hacked

1/4 cup red onion, finely hacked

1 lime, squeezed

2 tablespoons extra-virgin olive oil

1 teaspoon ground cumin

Salt and pepper to taste

Avocado cuts for embellish

Directions:

In a huge bowl, consolidate quinoa, dark beans, corn, red chime pepper, cilantro, and red onion.

In a little bowl, whisk together lime juice, olive oil, ground cumin, salt, and pepper.

Pour the dressing over the plate of mixed greens and throw to join.

Decorate with avocado cuts.

Serve chilled.

19. Fish and White Bean Salad

Fixings:

2 jars (5 oz every one) of canned fish in water, depleted

2 jars (15 oz each) of cannellini beans, depleted and flushed

1/2 cup cherry tomatoes, divided

1/4 cup red onion, finely cleaved

2 tablespoons new parsley, cleaved

2 tablespoons extra-virgin olive oil

1 tablespoon red wine vinegar

1 garlic clove, minced

Salt and pepper to taste

Guidelines:

In an enormous bowl, consolidate fish, cannellini beans, cherry tomatoes, red onion, and parsley.

In a little bowl, whisk together olive oil, red wine vinegar, minced garlic, salt, and pepper.

Pour the dressing over the plate of mixed greens and throw to join.

Serve chilled.

20. Spinach and Berry Salad

Fixings:

4 cups new child spinach leaves

1 cup blended berries (strawberries, blueberries, raspberries)

1/4 cup cleaved pecans

1/4 cup disintegrated goat cheddar

2 tablespoons balsamic vinegar

2 tablespoons extra-virgin olive oil

1 tablespoon honey

Salt and pepper to taste

Directions:

In an enormous serving of mixed greens bowl, join spinach, blended berries, cleaved pecans, and disintegrated goat cheddar.

In a little bowl, whisk together balsamic vinegar, olive oil, honey, salt, and pepper.

Sprinkle the dressing over the plate of mixed greens and throw to consolidate.

Serve right away.

21. Greek Tzatziki and Veggie Wrap

Fixings:

2 huge entire grain tortillas

1 cup Greek tzatziki sauce

1 cup cucumber, daintily cut

1 cup cherry tomatoes, split

1/2 cup red chime pepper, meagerly cut

1/4 cup red onion, daintily cut

1/4 cup new mint leaves

Salt and pepper to taste

Directions:

Spread out the tortillas and spread Greek tzatziki sauce equally over them.

Layer with cucumber cuts, cherry tomatoes, red chime pepper, and red onion.

Sprinkle new mint leaves on top.

Season with salt and pepper.

Roll up the tortillas firmly and cut down the middle askew.

Serve right away.

CONCLUSION

These no-cook supper recipes are heavenly as well as loaded with mitigating fixings to assist with advancing general wellbeing and prosperity. Enjoy!